Fertile Foundations

Mindful Pregnancy and Childbirth

Table of Contents

Chapter 1. Introduction

Introducing our new Special Report - "Fertile Foundations: Mindful Pregnancy and Childbirth." This enlightening guide serves as an essential companion for every woman considering or entering the beautiful journey towards motherhood. It sweeps across vital topics such as understanding fertility, the significance of mindful pregnancy, and the wonders of childbirth. It also explores modern approaches to prenatal care that seamlessly combine age-old wisdom with up-to-date medical insights. This special report is rich with expert guidance and practical tips, making it an indispensable resource for nurturing a healthy and joyful pregnancy experience. Exciting, isn't it? Wait till you unravel the insights awaiting inside. Come, let's embrace the miraculous journey of creation with grace, strength, and mindfulness!

Chapter 2. Understanding Fertility: Physiology and Cycles

Understanding fertility at a fundamental level is the first step on your path towards conscious parenthood. In essence, fertility is the natural capability to produce offspring. For most women, this is a cycle that repeats every month during their reproductive years, between puberty and menopause. However, understanding the nuances, timing, rhythms, and complexities of this cycle is imperative. This in-depth exploration will empower you with knowledge, aid in your family planning decisions, and enable a deeper connection with your body.

2.1. The Magic of the Female Reproductive System

The female reproductive system is an awe-inspiring wonder, capable of creating and nurturing life. It revolves around a handful of essential organs. The ovaries, fallopian tubes, uterus, and vagina each play a distinctive role in the conception and gestation process.

The ovaries hold your lifetime supply of eggs. Every month typically sees the release of a single mature egg, which then travels down the fallopian tubes in hopes of encountering sperm for fertilization. If this meeting occurs, the fertilized egg (now an embryo) continues on its journey to the uterus, where it implants into the uterine lining and begins the growth process.

2.2. The Menstrual Cycle: A Monthly Symphony of Hormones

The menstrual cycle is the monthly cycle of changes a woman's body goes through in preparation for the possibility of pregnancy. Each month, one of the ovaries releases an egg — a process called ovulation. At the same time, hormonal changes prepare the uterus for pregnancy. If ovulation takes place and the egg isn't fertilized, the lining of the uterus sheds through the vagina. This is a menstrual period.

The menstrual cycle, which is counted from the first day of one period to the first day of the next, isn't the same for every woman. Menstrual flow might occur every 21 to 35 days and last two to seven days.

2.3. Unpacking Ovulation

For most women trying to conceive, understanding ovulation is key. Ovulation refers to the monthly process by which a mature egg is released from one of your ovaries, setting the scene for possible conception. An egg survives for about 24 hours after release for fertilization by a sperm. In contrast, sperm can survive inside a woman for about 3-5 days. Therefore, pregnancy is technically possible from sexual intercourse that occurs at any time during the 5 days before ovulation and on the day of ovulation itself.

There are various signs and symptoms which indicate ovulation, including mid-cycle pain (mittelschmerz), a slight rise in basal body temperature, an increase in cervical mucus, and slight changes in the position and firmness of the cervix itself.

2.4. Fertility and Age: A Critical Correlation

While it's common knowledge that female fertility decreases with age, unpacking this correlation might help you make more informed reproductive decisions. Fertility usually starts to decline for women from about the age of 30, dropping down more steeply from the age of 35. As women grow older, not only does the quantity of potential eggs decrease, but the quality also diminishes, leading to lower chances of conception and higher chances of genetic abnormalities in the fetus.

2.5. The Role of Hormones

Hormones govern the processes of fertility and reproduction. The prominent ones include Follicle-Stimulating Hormone (FSH), Luteinizing Hormone (LH), estrogen, and progesterone. FSH and LH play critical roles in ovulation, with LH also aiding in the development of the corpus luteum. Estrogen helps prepare the uterus for pregnancy, but it also guides the release of LH and FSH during the menstrual cycle. After ovulation, progesterone works to maintain the uterine lining for implantation of an embryo.

2.6. Impact of Lifestyle on Fertility

Your lifestyle can greatly impact your fertility. Activities like smoking, overconsumption of alcohol, excessive caffeine intake, and the use of recreational drugs can negatively affect fertility. On the flip side, regular exercise, a balanced diet, managing stress, maintaining a healthy weight, avoiding exposure to harmful environmental factors, and stopping harmful habits like smoking can improve your fertility.

2.7. Understanding Infertility

While the word itself might sound disheartening, infertility is relatively common and is far from a hopeless condition. Infertility refers to not being able to get pregnant after one year of trying (or six months if a woman is 35 or older). Infertility can be due to a multitude of causes, and modern reproductive medicine now presents various treatments and procedures to overcome these hurdles.

Understanding your fertility is an important part of planning your family and caring for your reproductive health. This exploration has provided a comprehensive view of female fertility's physiological aspects, taking a deep dive into the menstrual cycle and the hormones that manage it, the role of age and lifestyle in fertility, and an overview of infertility. Armed with this information, you can embark on your journey towards motherhood with confidence and consciousness.

Chapter 3. Choosing the Right Time: Preconception Care and Planning

Choosing the right time to conceive bears significant implications on your physical and emotional well-being, as well as the health and development of your future child. Preconception care is a critical part of this process. By optimizing your health and addressing any potential risks before pregnancy, you empower yourself to have the healthiest pregnancy and childbirth possible.

3.1. Understanding Your Biological Clock

The concept of a "biological clock" has a basis in science, with research suggesting that fertility decreases over time, particularly for women. From birth, women possess a fixed number of eggs. The quality of these eggs deteriorates as one ages, making conception more challenging after certain ages - typically after the mid to late '30s and more dramatically after 40.

Understanding your biological clock isn't solely important for reasons of fertility. It also has implications for prenatal health and the health of your future child. Older parents may face higher risks of certain complications, including chromosomal disorders and miscarriages.

However, your biological clock isn't the only measure you need to consider. You must balance these factors with personal and lifestyle considerations - including your career, personal goals, and your relationship.

3.2. Preparing Your Body for Pregnancy

Preconception care also includes optimizing your physical health. Start by scheduling a preconception appointment with your healthcare provider to assess your health and address any concerns. This checkup should be based on your health history and lifestyle and might include the following:

- Comprehensive physical examination

- Blood tests to check for any existing conditions

- Update on immunizations

- Pap smear and pelvic exam

- Assessing any mental health concerns

Eating a balanced diet is crucial at this stage. Prenatal vitamins, especially those containing folic acid, are also important to prevent birth defects. Additionally, regular exercise can help you enter pregnancy at a healthy weight, which can reduce complications.

3.3. Lifestyle Changes for a Healthy Pregnancy

Lifestyles play a crucial role during conception and pregnancy. Smoking, alcohol, and drugs can affect fertility and can be harmful to a developing baby. If you smoke or drink alcohol, it's best to quit or at least limit your use before you become pregnant. Regular moderate exercise is also beneficial, as it helps to manage weight, boost mood, and strengthen your cardiovascular system, better preparing your body for the demands of pregnancy.

Getting enough sleep is just as essential. Studies suggest proper sleep can boost fertility and provide numerous health benefits.

3.4. The Mental Aspect: Stress and Conception

Numerous studies show a correlation between stress levels and fertility. High-stress levels might delay your ability to conceive and carry a pregnancy to term. The exact mechanisms of how stress impacts fertility remain a subject of ongoing research, but it seems wise to strive for a balanced, low-stress lifestyle when prepping for pregnancy.

Meditation, yoga, mindfulness, therapy, and other stress management techniques can help keep stress at bay. Also, consider creating a calm, nurturing environment where your future child will eventually live.

3.5. Tracking and Understanding Your Fertility Cycle

Understanding your fertility cycle can increase the chances of conception. The first day of your last menstrual period to the first day of your next period constitutes your menstrual cycle. Most women have a 28-day cycle; however, it's normal for this cycle to vary between 21 and 35 days.

Typically, ovulation occurs in the middle of your cycle, usually 14 days before your next period. This is when an egg is released from one of your ovaries, and it's the time when you're most fertile. Observing changes in your body, like your basal body temperature and cervical mucus, can help you identify when you're ovulating.

3.6. The Role of Preconception Genetic Screening

Preconception genetic screening can identify potential genetic disorders you and your partner might carry and pass on to your baby. This process is especially crucial if either of you has a family history of any inherited disorders, chromosomal disorders, or if certain genetic disorders are prevalent in your ethnic group.

3.7. Planning for Pregnancy: The Emotional Aspect

Emotionally preparing for pregnancy involves understanding and acknowledging the changes a baby brings. It's normal to feel a mixed range of emotions – happiness, anxiety, anticipation, and fear. Connect with your partner, share your feelings, and support each other during this phase. It may be worthwhile to connect with other parents-to-be or those who recently went through similar experiences.

Remember, choosing the right time for pregnancy is an intensely personal decision – one that's best made with plenty of thought and emotional preparation.

By devoting time to preconception care and planning, you're laying a strong and loving foundation for your future child. You're embarking on a wonderful journey, and these early steps can set the tone for what is to come – a satisfying, healthy, and joyful pregnancy and birth experience.

Chapter 4. The Mind-Body Connection in Pregnancy

To fully comprehend the mind-body connection in pregnancy, it is important to consider how these two systems, which are often discussed separately, are actually deeply intertwined and mutually influential.

4.1. The Physiology of the Mind-Body Connection

Our bodies and minds are in constant communication, forming a complex network of feedback loops that affect various aspects of our health and functioning. At the heart of the mind-body connection are the nervous and endocrine systems, which utilize hormones and neurotransmitters as their primary communication mechanisms.

During pregnancy, various physiological changes occur, with significant hormonal shifts that influence both the body and the mind. For example, hormones such as human chorionic gonadotrophin (hCG), progesterone, and estrogen surge during early pregnancy, promoting physical changes that accommodate the growing fetus and preparing the body for childbirth. These hormones also affect mood and cognitive function, leading to alterations in emotion and perception, known as pregnancy-specific brain changes.

Equally important are the neurochemicals produced by our minds in response to thoughts and feelings. Serotonin, dopamine, and oxytocin play vital roles in happiness, love, and well-being, and their levels may fluctuate during pregnancy. Understanding these interactions can help expectant mothers manage their emotions and maintain well-being throughout their journey.

4.2. Stress and Pregnancy: The Cortisol Connection

Among the factors that influence the mind-body interaction, stress holds a crucial role. Our body's response to stress is regulated by the hypothalamic-pituitary-adrenal (HPA) axis, which releases the hormone cortisol. Although cortisol is essential for regulating bodily functions, chronic stress can lead to excessive cortisol production, causing a cascade of potential problems, including inflammation, weight gain, and anxiety.

Pregnancy naturally induces a stress response in women, leading to an increase in cortisol levels. This elevation can support fetal development by promoting lung maturation but if left unchecked, it can affect the mind and body negatively. High cortisol levels during pregnancy can lead to increased risks of preterm birth and low birth weight and may affect the child's health and development later in life.

Becoming aware of stress triggers and learning stress-management techniques can help pregnant women maintain balanced cortisol levels. Techniques such as mindfulness, deep breathing, yoga, and meditation have been shown to reduce stress responses and promote a healthier pregnancy experience.

4.3. The Power of Positive Thinking: Neuroplasticity in Pregnancy

Our minds have an extraordinary capacity called neuroplasticity: the ability to form, strengthen, or weaken neural connections based on our thoughts, behaviors, and emotions. This concept implies that by focusing on positive thoughts and experiences, expectant mothers can wire their brains towards peace, positivity, and acceptance, which in turn can have beneficial effects on their bodies and their babies' health.

Even in pregnancy, the brain remains plastic and capable of adapting to change. Adjustments in thinking patterns can alter neural pathways, promoting better mood management, and healthier physiological responses to challenges. Practices that foster positivity, self-worth, and love can actively contribute to a mindful, enriched pregnancy experience.

4.4. Mindful Practices for a Harmonious Pregnancy

Understanding the mind-body connection allows us to respond mindfully to the dynamic changes pregnancy brings. Mindfulness, or the practice of being fully present in the moment, can help women navigate their pregnancy with less stress and more peace.

Mindful practices such as meditation, prenatal yoga, mindful eating, and listening to calming music can effectively boost serotonin and dopamine production while reducing cortisol levels. Furthermore, these practices can improve mental clarity, foster gratitude, and enhance the overall enjoyment of the pregnancy experience.

4.5. Visualization Techniques for a Positive Birthing Experience

Visualization, a powerful mind-body technique, involves creating vivid positive mental images. This practice can be particularly useful in preparing women for the birthing process. Visualizing a peaceful and successful delivery can instill confidence, reduce anxiety, and potentially influence labor's progression by promoting relaxation.

Birthing affirmations, a form of positive visualization, can also be a valuable psychological tool during labor. Repeating affirmations such as "My body is made to do this" or "Each wave brings me closer to meeting my baby" can offer emotional strength, encouraging women to trust in their bodies and the natural process of childbirth.

4.6. Postpartum Mind-Body Wellness

The mind-body connection continues to be an important factor after delivery. Postpartum is a time of intense change and adjustment, where hormonal shifts, fatigue, and emotional stress can take a toll on mental health. Guided relaxation, gentle exercise, and cognitive-behavioral techniques can support a new mother's wellbeing during this crucial period, proving the undeniable importance of attending to both mind and body.

Understanding and nurturing the mind-body connection can greatly enhance the pregnancy experience. By being mindful, practicing stress-reduction techniques, fostering positive thinking, and utilizing visualization, expectant mothers can foster an environment geared towards maximum wellbeing for both themselves and their babies. After all, pregnancy is not just about creating new life, but also about nurturing and affirming life already present within, by embracing the delicate balance of mind and body.

Chapter 5. Embracing Changes: Physical and Emotional Transformations

In the journey of pregnancy, your body becomes a nurturing home to a new life. This transformative process is marked with a series of physical and emotional changes that may leave you feeling thrilled, mystified, or sometimes overwhelmed. In this chapter, we'll walk you through these changes, helping you embrace them with understanding and respect.

5.1. Understanding Physical Changes

Pregnancy could be likened to an awe-inspiring orchestra, with numerous bodily functions playing in unison to create a unique symphony of life.

5.1.1. First Trimester Changes

In the first trimester, your body starts producing more hormones such as hCG (human chorionic gonadotropin), progesterone, and estrogen. This hormone surge often results in several physical changes.

- **Nausea and Vomiting:** Commonly known as morning sickness, this can occur at any time of the day due to a rise in hCG levels. Small, frequent meals and ginger-infused foods can help manage these symptoms.

- **Breast Tenderness:** Increased blood flow and hormonal changes might make your breasts sore, sensitive, or swollen. Supportive bras can help to alleviate discomfort.

- **Fatigue:** Your body is performing an energy-intensive task of creating another human, which can cause extreme tiredness.

5.1.2. Second Trimester Changes

In the second trimester, often regarded as the most comfortable period of pregnancy, substantial changes include:

- **Belly and Breast Growth:** Your expanding womb makes your belly more noticeable. Simultaneously, your breasts may continue to grow in preparation for breastfeeding.

- **Movement Sensations:** Around 20 weeks, you may begin to feel your baby's movements, initially resembling gentle flutters.

- **Skin Changes:** You might notice darkening of skin pigmentation around your nipples, a dark line down your belly (linea nigra), and stretch marks as your body expands.

5.1.3. Third Trimester Changes

By the third trimester, your body is on the home stretch, preparing for the forthcoming birth:

- **Braxton Hicks Contractions:** These "practice" contractions help your body get ready for real labor.

- **Shortness of Breath:** As your baby grows, your lungs have less space to expand, which can leave you feeling short of breath.

- **Swelling:** Fluid retention can lead to swollen feet and ankles. Regular movement and elevating your feet can help control this.

5.2. Embracing Emotional Changes

Alongside physical transformations, pregnancy often initiates a roller coaster of emotions.

5.2.1. Emotional Fluctuations

It's common to experience emotional highs and lows during pregnancy. These can be attributed to fluctuating hormone levels, changes in your body, and thoughts about impending motherhood.

Raised progesterone and estrogen levels can influence neurotransmitters, which might result in mood swings, anxiety, or depression. Ensure you discuss any strong emotional experiences with your healthcare provider.

5.2.2. Anticipatory Anxiety

Expecting a child brings excitement, but it's also natural to worry about the child's health, labor and delivery, or your abilities as a parent. Discussing these fears with your partner, a trusted friend, or a professional can provide a sense of comfort and preparedness.

5.2.3. Body Image Concerns

As your body transforms, coming to terms with your changing body image can be challenging. Remember, these changes are temporary and signify the incredible process your body is undergoing to nurture a new life. Be gentle with yourself.

5.3. Navigating the Changes

Embrace these changes as part and parcel of your miraculous journey towards motherhood.

5.3.1. Physical Self-care

Regular exercise, adequate rest, and a nutritious diet contribute to managing physical symptoms and promote overall well-being during pregnancy.

5.3.2. Emotional Self-Care

Mindfulness practices, journaling, and staying social can help manage emotional upheavals. There's no shame in seeking professional help if feelings of anxiety or depression persist.

Transformation implies change, and change takes time, patience, and understanding. By recognizing and embracing the physical and emotional shifts that occur with pregnancy, you're not just bearing a child, but evolving into the role of a mother. This is a dance of creation, where every step, every twirl, every heartbeat is a sign of the life forming within you. And you, dear mother, are the beautiful and resilient cradle in which this dance unfolds.

Awareness, understanding, and support can make this metamorphosis less daunting and more empowering. So, let's celebrate the changes, respect our bodies, mind, and emotions, and walk this journey with grace, strength, and love.

Chapter 6. The Power of Nutrition: Eating for Two

Every journey towards motherhood begins with the recognition that you're not just eating for yourself anymore. Each bite becomes a direct offering to the little life blossoming inside you. As such, nutrition takes precedence. What you eat directly influences the development and growth of your baby, significantly impacting their health later in life. Hence, understanding the power of nutrition is vital.

6.1. Understanding Pregnancy Nutrition

Pregnancy nutrition is not just about eating more. It involves consuming the right elements, in the right proportions. It's a delicate symbiosis of proteins, carbohydrates, fats, vitamins, and minerals that serve as the building blocks for your baby's development.

One fundamental principle of pregnancy nutrition is balance - ensuring that you have a diverse diet that covers various nutrients. An ideal plate should be brimming with vibrant colors, each representing different food groups. Incorporate a variety of vegetables, fruits, lean proteins, whole grains, and dairy products.

6.2. Nutrient Needs During Pregnancy

Certain nutrients become even more crucial during pregnancy. Here are some of them:

• Folic Acid: An essential nutrient right from the start, folic acid helps minimize the risk of neural tube defects in your baby. Fortified cereals, leafy greens, and citrus fruits are high in folic acid.

- Iron: Your body requires double the amount of iron to make hemoglobin for increasing blood volume. Iron-rich foods include lean meat, poultry, spinach, and iron-fortified cereals.

- Calcium: For the baby's bone development, adequate calcium intake is necessary. Include sources like dairy products, tofu, almonds, and broccoli in your diet.

- Protein: The building block of the body, protein is vital for your baby's growth, especially in the second and third trimester. Include lean meats, poultry, fish, eggs, beans, tofu, cheese, milk, seeds, and nuts in your diet.

- Fiber: To avoid problems like constipation and hemorrhoids that are common in pregnancy, include fiber-rich foods in your meals such as whole grains, legumes, fruits, and vegetables.

While supplements can provide some of these nutrients, the primary source should be a properly balanced diet. Always consult your healthcare provider before starting any supplement regime.

6.3. Specific Dietary Recommendations

Let's delve deeper into what your daily meals should look like during pregnancy:

1. Carbohydrates: Aim for whole grain choices, providing you with the necessary energy and aiding in digestion.

2. Proteins: Include lean meat, poultry, fish, eggs, or plant-based proteins like lentils, chickpeas, and tofu.

3. Fruits and Vegetables: Try to "eat the rainbow," meaning include

fruits and vegetables of different colors to your meals.

4. Dairy: Opt for low-fat or non-fat dairy products to supply necessary calcium and vitamin D.

Remember, your calorie intake will increase as your pregnancy advances and based on your pre-pregnancy weight, physical activity, and metabolism.

6.4. Foods to Avoid

While discussing what to include, it's equally important to remember foods to avoid or consume with caution:

- Unpasteurized Dairy and Juices: These contain harmful bacteria like Listeria that could harm you and your baby.

- High Mercury Fish: Certain sea foods are high in mercury, which isn't good for your baby's developing brain.

- Alcohol: Alcohol gets directly passed to your baby and can affect their development.

- Caffeine: High levels of caffeine can increase the risk of miscarriage or preterm birth. Limit your intake.

- Undercooked or Raw Foods: They can carry harmful bacteria and parasites.

Discuss with your healthcare provider about the foods you need to limit or avoid.

6.5. Sailing Through Morning Sickness

Morning sickness is a common pregnancy ailment that can often hinder optimal nutrition. Taking small frequent meals, not lying down immediately after meals, opting for bland foods over spicy or greasy ones, and ginger or lemon can often help. Stay hydrated and rest enough to manage the symptoms.

6.6. Staying Hydrated

Adequate hydration is as significant as nutritious meals. You need extra fluids to support the increase in your blood volume. Water remains the best choice, but you can also hydrate with decaffeinated teas, fruit-infused water, or low-sugar beverages.

Remember, each pregnancy is unique, and so are the dietary needs. With this comprehensive guide, ensure you nourish your body and pave the way for a healthy pregnancy. However, individual needs may vary, thereby underlining the importance of personal consultations with healthcare professionals who can offer diet recommendations based on specific requirements. Because at the end of the day, it's not just about eating for two, it's about eating right for two.

With every step of this beautiful motherhood journey, remember, you are creating life, and what could be more powerful than that! May the power of nutrition guide you delicately on this path!

Chapter 7. Staying Active: Safe Exercise During Pregnancy

While pregnancy is a time of great physical and emotional change, it is also an opportunity to establish practices that will help maintain wellness and fortify the connection with your growing baby. Exercise, when conducted mindfully and safely, can dramatically ameliorate some of the common discomforts of pregnancy such as leg cramps, fatigue, and backaches and can possibly simplify labor and delivery, and recovery postpartum.

However, the type, duration, and intensity of the exercise will depend on several factors including the stage of your pregnancy, your overall health, and your fitness level prior to becoming pregnant.

7.1. Understand why Exercise is Important

Engaging in regular physical activity while pregnant provides many health benefits. These include improved cardiovascular function, healthy weight management, enhanced strength and stamina for labor, improved mood, increased energy levels, and faster recovery post-childhood.

Moreover, remaining active and maintaining a fitness routine can also alleviate symptoms like nausea and morning sickness, improve sleep, promote muscle tone, strength, and endurance and can potentially reduce complications such as gestational diabetes, preeclampsia, and caesarean delivery.

7.2. Know Your Limits

The first rule of prenatal workouts is to listen to your body. If you're feeling poorly, overly tired, or experiencing any sort of pain, it's absolutely okay to take a rest day. Be aware of unusual symptoms such as persistent shortness of breath, dizziness, vaginal bleeding, chest pain, or any form of discomfort during pregnancy. If you notice any of these, consult your doctor immediately.

Bear in mind that every pregnant body reacts differently to exercise. Thus, it's crucial not to compare your fitness or strength levels with others. Remember, the overarching goal of exercise during pregnancy is overall wellness rather than setting personal records or achieving drastic physical transformations.

7.3. Choose the Right Exercises

There are many types of exercises that can be safely performed during pregnancy. Here are a few you might consider:

1. Walking: This is one of the safest forms of exercise during pregnancy and can be easily incorporated into daily routines.

2. Swimming: This exercise works many different parts of the body without adding strain and discomfort. The feeling of weightlessness in the water can be extremely comforting.

3. Prenatal Yoga: This exercise focuses on the connection of breath and movements, good for relieving tension and promoting relaxation. Always ensure you are supervised by a certified prenatal yoga instructor.

4. Prenatal Pilates: It assists in maintaining good posture, strengthens core muscles, and enhances overall body strength.

5. Low-impact Aerobics: This type of exercise helps maintain a healthy heart while keeping your muscles toned without causing

undue stress on your joints.

Always exercise with care, avoiding any rapid changes in your body's direction that might make you feel dizzy.

7.4. Gear up Right

Wearing comfortable, loose-fitting clothes while exercising is essential. A good supportive bra can make workouts more comfortable. Wear appropriate footwear designed specifically for the type of workout you are doing, providing adequate support and cushioning. Keep a bottle of water handy at all times to prevent dehydration.

7.5. Optimal Nutrition for Active Moms

Eating a nutritious diet is vital during pregnancy, and even more so when combined with regular exercise. The diet should include plenty of proteins, carbohydrates, and healthy fats needed for energy while working out. A diet rich in fruits, vegetables, lean proteins, and whole grains will support both your health and the development of the baby. Hydration is also of prime importance both during and after workouts.

7.6. Cooling Down and Stretching

Just as a warm-up is essential to prepare your body for exercise, a cool-down period is important to slowly bring your body back to its normal state. Include a 5-10 minutes cool-down period after your workout. Finish off with gentle stretching exercises to improve flexibility and reduce muscle soreness.

Remember to take it slowly and make sure every movement is

controlled and smooth to help prevent injury.

Staying active during pregnancy is an investment in overall health and well-being for both mom and baby. It can enable moms-to-be to better handle the physical demands of pregnancy, labor, and becoming a new mom. Adopt a more mindful approach to your exercise routine – one that listens to your body and respects its changing needs. Your body is, after all, in the process of performing a miraculous feat: nurturing and carrying a new life within!

Always remember to consult your healthcare provider before making any significant changes to your exercise routine during pregnancy. They can guide and make recommendations based on your medical history, current health status, and unique needs during this special time.

Chapter 8. Preparing for the Big Day: Understanding Childbirth

Understanding childbirth – the moment that crowns the journey of pregnancy – requires a comprehensive approach towards various dimensions including the basics of childbirth, the changes that pregnancy brings, stages of labor, pain relief measures, potential complications, and the role of partners during labor. Delving into each of these elements will help us prepare better for the big day.

8.1. The Basics of Childbirth

Childbirth is a natural process usually occurring around 40 weeks after the last menstrual period. It involves a harmonious play of hormones, especially oxytocin and endorphins, which kick starts contractions leading to the delivery of the baby. There are three ways of giving birth: vaginal delivery, cesarean-section (c-section), and vaginal birth after cesarean (VBAC). While vaginal delivery is the most common type, a c-section might be required under certain medical circumstances. VBAC is a viable option for women who've previously undergone a c-section, but with its own set of requirements and risks.

8.2. Pregnancy and Body Changes

Pregnancy ushers a whole host of changes in a woman's body. Hormonal imbalances could cause morning sickness, fatigue, and mood swings. The body accommodates the growing baby by enlarging the abdomen, leading to changes in the center of gravity and potential back pain. Breasts become larger and tender in preparation for breastfeeding. Frequent urination, constipation, and heartburn are common due to hormonal changes and mechanical pressure exerted by the growing uterus.

8.3. Understanding Stages of Labor

Labor, leading to childbirth, typically unfolds in three stages:

1. First Stage: This is the longest stage commenced by contractions and characterized by effacement (thinning out) and dilation (opening of) the cervix.

2. Second Stage: This stage involves pushing and birth of the baby.

3. Third Stage: Also known as afterbirth, this involves the delivery of the placenta.

8.4. Pain Relief Measures

Labor induces pain due to contractions and stretching of tissues. Several pain relief measures exist, ranging from non-pharmacological methods like mobility during labor, hydrotherapy, massage, and relaxation techniques, to pharmacological measures like epidural analgesia, nitrous oxide, and opioid medications. The choice depends on the mother's comfort and the medical team's recommendation.

8.5. Potential Complications

While childbirth is a natural process, it may sometimes present complications. These range from minor deviations from the normal course of labor like slow progression of labor, to serious issues like fetal distress, umbilical cord issues, or maternal complications. Understanding the potential complications is crucial for maintaining the health of mother and baby.

8.6. The Role of Partners During Labor

Partners play a significant role in childbirth. Their presence and support provide emotional strength to the pregnant woman during labor. They can assist by providing comfort, encouragement, and helping with pain relief methods.

Understanding childbirth is a multidimensional process with a series of physical and emotional changes leading to the momentous event of welcoming the new member in the family. It might seem daunting, but with knowledge comes empowerment. Knowing what to expect and how to cope offers a sense of control and confidence, making the beautiful journey towards childbirth a cherished experience filled with joy and anticipation.

Chapter 9. Prenatal Care Choices: Making Informed Decisions

Understanding the importance of well-guided prenatal care is your first step in welcoming the life you are about to create. In essence, prenatal care is the optimum health management and wellness promotion approach designed for you and your future baby.

9.1. Understanding Prenatal Care

Prenatal care encompasses regular doctor's visits and lifestyle changes to ensure both mother and baby's health. It can begin even before pregnancy, known as **preconception care**, transitioning into **prenatal care** during pregnancy, and concluded with **postpartum care** after childbirth.

Prenatal care aims to spot health problems early, prevent complications, and educate expectant mothers about pregnancy to childbirth. It touches upon the physical, emotional, and spiritual aspects of the mother. Building a strong foundation with prenatal care contributes to successful birth deliveries and healthy babies.

Several studies show a strong correlation between consistent prenatal care and decreased rates of maternal and infant mortality. Furthermore, it improves the mother's mental health by reducing stress, anxiety, and depression during pregnancy.

9.2. Choosing Your Prenatal Care Provider

Different types of health professionals can provide prenatal care. They include obstetricians (OB-GYNs), family physicians, certified nurse-midwives, maternity care providers, perinatologists, etc. Your choice will depend on your health status, personal preferences, belief system, and the type of birth experience you desire.

OB-GYNs are doctors who specialize in pregnancy and childbirth. They are skilled in managing medical complications in both mother and baby, including surgery (caesarean section).

Family physicians are doctors who provide general health care. Some can also take care of low-risk pregnancies and deliveries.

Certified Nurse-Midwives are registered nurses with special training in prenatal care, childbirth, postpartum, and routine gynecological care. They assist uncomplicated pregnancies typically focusing on a holistic approach with less medical intervention.

Perinatologists or Maternal-Fetal Medicine Specialists cater to high-risk pregnancies, complicated health issues, and special-needs infants.

You might choose to have a team of professionals to ensure all-around care. Each can contribute uniquely to your pregnancy experience.

9.3. Prenatal Testing

Prenatal tests are essential components of prenatal care. They ensure the baby's health and monitor the progress of the pregnancy.

Prenatal testing includes both screening tests and diagnostic tests.

Screening tests indicate the possibility of a particular condition. Common screening tests include ultrasound, quad marker screen, etc.

Diagnostic tests confirm the presence of a specific condition. These include Amniocentesis or Chorionic Villus Sampling.

Not all tests are needed for every woman. The tests required will depend on factors such as age, health status, family history, ethnic background, etc. Discuss with your provider to determine which tests are best for you.

9.4. Prenatal Nutrition and Lifestyle Management

Maintaining a healthy lifestyle and diet is pivotal during pregnancy.

Your diet should be rich in fiber, protein, calcium, fruits, and vegetables. Hydration is also crucial. A balanced diet promotes proper fetal development. Seek guidance from your care provider or a nutritionist to build a diet plan tailored to you.

An active lifestyle contributes to easier pregnancy and childbirth. Simple exercises such as walking, swimming, or prenatal yoga can help. However, always consult with your healthcare provider before starting an exercise regimen.

Additionally, meditation and stress management techniques should be integrated. These practices enhance emotional health, contributing to overall wellness.

Avoid harmful substances like alcohol, tobacco, and drugs. These can lead to severe complications such as premature birth, developmental issues, and infant mortality.

9.5. Prenatal Education

Prenatal education serves as a tool to prepare for childbirth and parenthood. They enlighten about labor, birth, breastfeeding, newborn care, and postpartum adjustments. You can access prenatal education through classes, books, online platforms, etc., based on convenience and comfort.

Making informed decisions and actively participating in your care enriches your pregnancy journey. It emphasizes the importance of prenatal care, which is not merely a series of exams and pulses-checking sessions but a comprehensive approach vital in envisioning and realizing a healthy and joyful motherhood. Learning is an integral part of this journey as every mother carves her unique path in this shared experience.

There is a wave of changes when stepping into parenthood. Good prenatal care choices support and guide as you harness this wave into a transformative journey, embracing the beautiful process of birthing life.

Chapter 10. Reducing Pregnancy Concerns: Overcoming Common Hurdles

Pregnancy is a time of great joy but also of concern and worry to many prospective mothers. Not knowing what to expect, the physical changes, or the myriad of possible complications can be daunting. However, with good knowledge and understanding, most concerns can be effectively managed or even mitigated.

10.1. Understanding and Mitigating Morning Sickness

Morning sickness, characterized by nausea and vomiting, is one of the most common concerns during early pregnancy affecting around 70 percent of pregnant women. Despite its name, it can occur at any time throughout the day or night. The primary cause is believed to be the rapid increase in human chorionic gonadotropin (hCG) hormone soon after conception. This nausea usually begins around the sixth week of pregnancy and often subsides by the fourteenth week.

To manage morning sickness:

1. Eat small meals to avoid an empty stomach.

2. Avoid foods and smells that make your nausea worse.

3. Drink lots of water to stay hydrated – dehydration can make nausea worse.

4. Eat a snack, such as dry toast or crackers, before getting out of bed in the morning.

Despite the discomfort, morning sickness often indicates a healthy pregnancy. However, severe morning sickness, or hyperemesis gravidarum, can require medical attention as it can lead to severe dehydration and weight loss.

10.2. Managing Fatigue

Your body works hard growing a new life, and this can result in fatigue. This is completely normal, particularly in the early stages of pregnancy and then again in the final trimester. Rest and a balanced diet can combat fatigue:

1. Establish a regular sleep routine.

2. Include physical activity, such as a light walk, in your daily routine.

3. Stay hydrated and consume a diet high in protein and complex carbohydrates.

10.3. Tackling Back Pain

Back pain during pregnancy, commonly in the lower back, is often due to changes in your body's alignment. Extra weight, changes in posture, as well as hormone changes, contribute to this problem. To help alleviate this pain:

1. Ensure proper posture when sitting or standing.

2. Engage in exercises such as walking or prenatal yoga for strengthening and stretching your muscles.

3. Avoid lifting heavy objects.

Remember to always consult your medical practitioner before beginning any exercise routines.

10.4. Coping with Changes in Body Image

Pregnancy causes many physical changes that might impact your body image and self-esteem. Weight gain, darkening of skin (melasma), stretch marks, and changes to your shape are all perfectly normal.

Maintain a positive perspective towards these changes as they are signs of the incredible work your body is doing to prepare for your baby's arrival.

10.5. Dealing with Emotional Rollercoaster

Besides physical changes, pregnancy can come with an emotional whirlwind due to hormonal changes. This fluctuation of emotions might result in mood swings.

To keep your emotional wellness:

1. Communicate your feelings with your partner, loved ones, or a mental health professional.
2. Engage in stress-reducing activities such as leisure walks, meditation, or prenatal yoga.
3. Maintain adequate rest and follow a balanced diet.

Know that it's okay not to be constantly overjoyed during your pregnancy. If feelings of depression or anxiety persist, reach out to a healthcare professional without delay.

10.6. Prepping for Labour and Delivery

The thought of labour and delivery can be intimidating. Remember, your body is designed to carry and birth a baby, and medical advances have made it safer than ever.

To alleviate fears:

1. Attend prenatal classes.

2. Establish a birth plan that includes your wishes for your birthing experience.

3. Stay informed about the stages of labour and delivery process.

Ultimately, every pregnancy is unique, and it's important to remain patient with your body, stay informed, and keep an open line of communication with your healthcare provider. As you prepare to welcome your new child, remember that it's okay to have concerns. Knowledge and understanding will help you make the best decisions for your health and for the health of your baby. You're embarking on one of life's most beautiful journeys – enjoy the ride.

Chapter 11. Postpartum Journey: From Recovery to Bonding

The moments following childbirth bring an array of unique experiences ranging from physical changes to emotional shifts, all the way to the bonding process with your newborn. The focus of this chapter is to navigate you through this important stage of your motherhood journey, making the transition as smooth as possible.

11.1. Understanding Postpartum Recovery

Generally, the postpartum period encompasses the first six weeks following childbirth. In light of the significant changes your body undergoes during this time, the process of recovery may be more complex and longer than you might anticipate.

Physical recovery poses the immediate challenge after delivery. Whether you've had a vaginal delivery or a C-section, your body needs time to heal. During the first week, you may experience contractions as your uterus returns to its usual size. Common symptoms such as postpartum bleeding (lochia) and perineum soreness can last several weeks. A C-section recovery may include pain at the site of the incision and in the abdomen, impairment of bowel movements, and mood swings.

Apart from physical aspects, the early postpartum phase is also characterized by hormonal fluctuations leading to emotional changes. About 50-80% of new mothers experience 'baby blues', characterized by mood swings, crying spells, anxiety, and difficulty sleeping, usually a few days after childbirth. This is a normal response to the dramatic hormone changes and the challenges of taking care of a newborn.

However, if these feelings persist longer than two weeks and become more intense, it may signal postpartum depression (PPD). PPD requires attention and treatment from health care professionals. Also, don't hesitate to ask for psychological support if it becomes overwhelming.

Moreover, the demands linked to the new role — lack of sleep and frequent feeding — can lead to exhaustion. Add potential breastfeeding issues to the mix and it becomes obvious how critical postpartum care is.

Taking care of your physical well-being, addressing emotional changes, identifying when to seek help, and allowing yourself enough time to heal are all vital elements of recovery.

11.2. Nourishment and Self-Care

Eating a balanced diet contributes significantly to physical recovery and supports the additional energy needed for breastfeeding. You need an estimated 500 extra calories per day if you're nursing.

A varied diet with protein, whole grains, fruits, vegetables, and healthy fats provides the necessary vitamins and minerals. Also, consider discussing the need for any supplements with a healthcare provider.

Collaboration is crucial at this stage. Welcome help from supportive loved ones or engage a postpartum doula if accessible. Make sure to guard your sleep as best you can. Done in shifts, caring for the baby allows you some restorative hours of sleep.

11.3. Bonding with Your Baby

Extraordinary as birth is, the bonding process between you and your newborn is equally magical. While some mothers feel an instant connection with their babies, for others, this bond takes a little more time to develop. Both learn to understand and communicate with each other during this first connection phase.

Breastfeeding can be a valuable bonding time. The skin-to-skin contact releases 'the bonding hormone' oxytocin for both you and your baby, fostering a strong bond of love and trust.

Engage in activities that involve close contact, such as baby massage or simply carrying your baby against your chest. These small moments of interaction strengthen the connection.

Communication through eyes and voices, responding to the baby's cues, understanding your baby's individual schedule, and maintaining a calm presence enhance the bonding process.

11.4. Challenges along the Postpartum Road

Despite it being a time of joy, the postpartum journey can sometimes feel overwhelming when faced with challenges that you might not have anticipated.

Breastfeeding is a naturally beautiful experience but it is also a skill that needs to be learned by both mother and baby, which may come with challenges. If you run into issues like insufficient lactation, painful nursing, or if your baby is having trouble latching on, don't hesitate to seek advice from a lactation consultant or your healthcare provider.

Furthermore, the risk of postpartum depression should not be overlooked. Be alert for feelings of persistent sadness or anxiety, changes in sleeping or eating patterns, and problems focusing or making decisions. Don't hesitate to seek professional help if these feelings surface.

Always remember to be kind to yourself during this journey, and understand that it's okay to seek help when needed. This time is filled with natural ups and downs, and every mother has her own unique experience.

11.5. Conclusion

The postpartum journey is filled with a variety of experiences from healing, adjusting to a new life rhythm, bonding with your newborn, and even overcoming challenges. It's a phase to be cherished, knowing you're not alone in the journey, and that support is accessible whenever required. Ensure that you give yourself the time and care you need during this special period as you and your baby begin to develop a lifetime bond.

Remember, while guidance and advice are handy, listen to your inner voice and trust your own instincts too. You are your baby's first love, and this journey, with all its experiences, is the beginning of many more beautiful beginnings to come. No mother's journey is the same, and each experience is as unique as you are. Cherish it, embrace it.